CW00408423

# The Power of Walking

## The 30 Day Plan that shows you how to get moving again

IAN BIRCH

Copyright © 2023 Ian Birch

All rights reserved. No part of this book may be reproduced or transmitted in any form or by any means, electronic or mechanical, including photocopying, recording, or by any information storage and retrieval system by anyone but the purchaser for their own personal use. This book may not be reproduced in any form without the express written permission of Ian Birch prior to publication.

ISBN: 979-8850740658

# DISCLAIMERS

**Always consult your doctor**. If you are in any doubt regarding your health, then consult your doctor before making any changes to your lifestyle including exercise or diet, and follow their advice.

**The information presented in this book is for educational purposes only.** This should not replace advice from a qualified medical professional and does not offer medical advice as I am not a medical doctor. The information in this book is based on my own personal experiences and on my own interpretation of research and other available sources.

**This book is for healthy adults.** The information in this book is intended for healthy adults. If you have any concerns regarding your health, you must consult your doctor and follow their advice.

**This book does not offer guaranteed outcomes.** The book describes outcomes Ian Birch experienced personally. The outcomes for anyone following the suggested exercises will vary for many reasons and so the outcomes cannot be guaranteed. Ian Birch does not assume liability for any injuries, personal loss, or illness caused by the use of this information.

**Keep this fun and enjoyable.** It is the intention of the author to provide a fitness plan that is easy to adapt to just about any individual lifestyle. The author found that making exercise fun and enjoyable played an important part of his own successful outcomes and encourages you to do the same.

# CONTENTS

# ACKNOWLEDGMENTS

I must start by saying thank you to my family for their encouragement for me to put pen to paper and for their ongoing support to complete what turned out to be a larger task than first appeared.

I must also thank my good friend Alan Watson, otherwise known as "Alan the Artist" for his numerous sketches that livened up the original notes and some of which now live on in the final work.

Finally, I would like to thank the various sources I have used to illustrate important points or provide various data or concepts. And I will finish by stating that any errors, mistakes or omissions are mine and mine alone.

# 1. WHO SHOULD READ THIS BOOK

This book is written for anyone trying to get moving and trying to build activity into their lives. It doesn't matter if you were super fit back in the day or if you are trying to start exercising for the first time. You may be younger, say 30s or 40s, or a bit older 50s and 60s (like me).

You really want to do something about this now because it isn't just about your fitness anymore. It's not just about losing some excess weight either. This is much bigger. This is about your health, your wellbeing, your life even!

As I struggled to find a way to reclaim my own health & fitness, I had this driven feeling. Yes, I wanted to trim my bulging waist, but more importantly:

## "I needed to get moving again because I wanted my life back"

But you may well have already tried to get active and stumbled just like I did so many times. So you might be asking yourself the same questions like:

## "Why is this so hard?
### or
## Why can't I make this work?"

And maybe you feel like there are some sort of impossible hurdles or barriers that just seem to bring every attempt to a grinding halt, despite all your best efforts.

If this sound familiar, well I can tell you that there is something else going on. There were genuine reasons why I kept failing and these could be holding you back too.

For one thing, my body wasn't ready to move the way I expected and wanted it to and I'll come back to this a little later. But this did explain why going back to old training protocols and methods just didn't work.

I found this difficult to come to terms with at first and you might too.

But if you can accept that your body isn't quite ready to move the way you want it to just yet, then you can take a different journey back to health and fitness too.

Look, the human body is designed to move. Movement is important for our health as well as our fitness. **We are designed to move!**

And *The Power of Walking* can help just about anyone to get moving again.

This short book gives you a *30 Day Plan* to help break through the barriers holding you back and change your direction of travel. It will show you:

- Why movement is important for both your health and your fitness.
- How to build simple exercise habits into your life
- How to get the absolute most from the exercise of walking
- How to use the 30 days as a springboard to an active life

But it's much more than that because this *30 Day Plan* shows you how to use the most natural and fundamental human movement of walking to start training like an athlete. Now your regular exercise can be invigorating rather than exhausting so you can make it a fun and enjoyable part of your new lifestyle.

Stick to the plan and you will start making little gains. You may not notice them at first, but they are there. And these gains keep getting a little bit bigger until finally you realise that you are up and running.

Once you are moving again, you can start reclaiming your health & fitness. And then you might even look to take on a bigger challenge like:

- "10,000 Steps a Day" or "Couch to 5k"
- Joining a local walking group to go hiking.
- Joining a running group like Park Run
- Re-joining your old sports club
- Signing up at the Gym to start Weight Training again.

Or maybe you just want to get active again to help you:

- Lose some weight.
- Regain your energy and feel more alert.
- Just do some of the things you used to love doing.
- Look great for a big occasion like a wedding or special holiday.

When I started walking again everything changed. Now you can use the same plan to get moving too. And in just 30 days you could be ready to tackle whatever it is that inspires you. But the most important thing is to start, so go on:

## Start walking to reclaim your health & fitness

And whatever you decide, I hope this brief introduction will still encourage you to start walking to get movement back into your life. You've got to know that you can do this. You can get active, and it is just so worth it.

# 2. MY PROMISE TO YOU

Look I get it, you want to do something about your fitness and deep down you know you have to. You might even have tried to do something already, maybe trying to start walking or running, even joining a gym or fitness class. But you just couldn't make it work and now it's gone again. It's not just life getting in the way, something else is going on.

But now this is bigger. This isn't just about fitness anymore, is it? This is about more than your health too. In fact, this is about your life, the people dear to you, being strong for your family and friends. Grabbing your life back even.

Now, what if I can help explain why getting active again can be so tough for so many of us. And then show you a way to start exercising regularly at a level just about anybody can manage.

The tell-tale sign is your waist. A bulging waist can indicate an increasing risk of serious diseases, in other words deteriorating health. It can also indicate how far your strength and fitness have fallen. And that is why it can be so tough to get moving again.

So I want to show you a way to start exercising that just about anyone can manage. What's more, it is really effective and so flexible it can fit into just about any lifestyle. It can help you start losing that waistline bulge, start regaining your energy and rekindle that feeling that you can take on the world again.

And it doesn't matter how unfit you are, if you can walk you can do this. Still, I understand if you find it hard to believe that you can turn your health & fitness around just walking. But there is a secret in *The Power of Walking* that we can all take advantage of and using this secret we can start training like an athlete.

If you take on the challenge and commit to follow the plan for the 30 days then I have to warn you that your fitness will only come back slowly at first.

And I should also warn you that you might lose some weight, but it isn't going to suddenly drop off. In fact, I suggest that rather than tracking your weight, you will find it more useful to track your waistline. I'll explain why shortly.

But as I also will explain, you are rebuilding the very foundations of your fitness and health all over again. And if you can accept where you are physically right now and if you trust the process, the gains will start.

Those gains are more than just physical. Your mindset can start to shift as you learn to value your health and fitness again. Just getting out and about opens your eyes to your surroundings and you might see views for the first time or enjoy the birds that you've never really noticed before.

And you will also find that training smart like an athlete doesn't exhaust you, it invigorates you.

You just can't wait to move onto the next level but at the same time you won't feel inclined to rush into it.

You're more likely to enjoy the satisfaction of steadily reclaiming your health and fitness all over again, one step at a time.

So I'm not promising that you're going to turn your health and fitness completely around in a mere 30 days. But I can promise that you can change your direction of travel right around and make exercise an essential part of your life again. Then you can start to enjoy all the benefits that flow from that.

And you just never know where this journey might lead you.

I mean when I set out on 1st Nov 2013, I did not expect to be a fully operational firefighter 7 months later or to get back in a racing eight or take up OCR.

But all these happened because I just got started and I started with brisk walking.

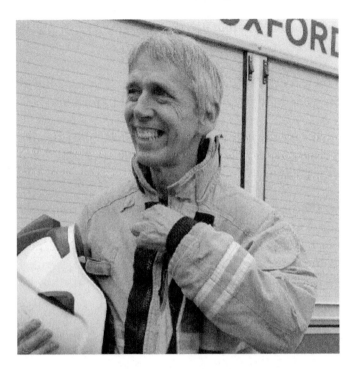

**Fig 1. The Accidental Firefighter**

**Where will your journey take you?**

# 3. WHO AM I AND WHY I WROTE THIS BOOK

Well, I should have written this book back in 2013/14 because that is when I first used this simple but effective plan. Let me explain.

My 55th birthday was looming into view and I realised that my fitness was shot but worse still my health was failing.

I hadn't been ill as such for some years, but I was just tired all the time. I had been monitoring my weight and I was only maybe 5-6 pounds overweight.

Even though my BMI Score was still "healthy" I knew something wasn't right because I had somehow changed to a horrible, skinny fat shape now.

The bulge around my waist had become very noticeable so I finally calculated my Waist to Height Ratio.

Now the universal indicator is a measure of 0.5. Below this and you are in good shape. Above this and you are heading into high health risk territory.

I got a real shock, mine was now well over 0.52. and I was now into high-risk territory for a host of unpleasant diseases like Heart Attack, High Blood Pressure and Diabetes.

I finally had to acknowledge that I had a health problem as well as a fitness problem.

As all this was going on through the first half of 2013, I tried some old training methods I had used years before. But each time I just broke down.

With each failure I got more and more down, thinking that was it, I was just past it and destined to get old early.

But I was familiar with the science backing up *The Power of Walking.* I knew all about how elite athletes train to their metabolic levels. Heck, I had coached loads of junior rowing athletes. Some had never trained in any sport before, and my message had always been the same:

## **Accept where you are, train to your metabolic levels and then let the magic happen.**

The Juniors loved it. They trained to their metabolic bands and just piled on the fitness and got noticeably leaner.

I even ended up writing short programmes for some of the parents because they had seen how well it was working and they wanted to get the same benefits.

Some wanted to get fitter and some wanted to trim some excess weight.

Reflecting back to early 2013 and my various attempts to get moving again I had to admit to myself that I had failed to take heed of that very first step in the process.

But now I was ready to:

## Accept where I was
## and that the only exercise
## I could manage was a brisk walk.

I finally accepted that my strength and fitness had declined more than I cared to admit before.

In other words, I finally accepted "Where I Was Now" and tested my walking to see if it really could work. It did, so as autumn 2013 came around I put together my little plan.

And I should point out that I didn't just want to get moving again, I also wanted to get out and about again. I wanted to get out in the fresh air to start feeling alive again.

So I found some pleasant walking routes including the path in **Fig 2** over the page which I still frequent to this day.

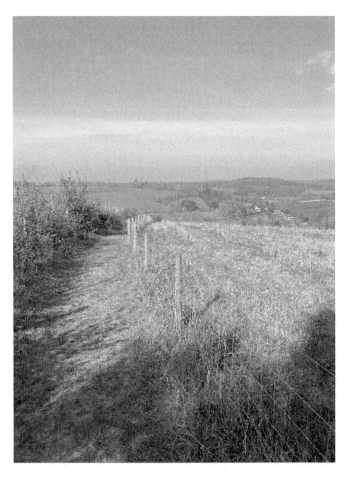

**Fig 2. Getting Out into the Countryside**

## 3.1. My First 30 Days

So, when I started on 1st Nov 2013:

- I already knew that I could walk briskly for 20-25 mins.
- I already had a clear understanding of how to train at my metabolic levels.
- And I knew deep down that training at the right metabolic level should work even though it does feel counterintuitive.

My overall plan mapped out a progression over 90 Days.

But I was very conscious that I had to let my body ease into this new pattern of exercise. Something I had failed to do in the past.

And so the first month, or rather my First 30 Days, was dedicated to just walking.

I set aside three times a week on a weekly planner and tested out a few walking routes.

In each session I would make my way to the start of one of my routes and complete a 20-25 walk at the pace I needed to.

That was my time, no distractions. I might only be walking but as far as I was concerned, I was training again.

## 3.2. And the Results

I must admit that I was genuinely surprised by some outcomes:

- I found that I enjoyed the sessions and looked forward to them.
- I found the sessions invigorating and felt like I was getting a little faster and a little looser.
- I might have lost a pound or two. Not enough to be really noticeable.
- BUT I had definitely lost an inch around the waist.

In fact, I couldn't quite believe the waist measurement. I kept checking it over and over for a few days. But it kept coming up the same:

## I had lost the first inch from my waistline

## 3.3 My Big Breakthrough (at last)

In fact, by day 30 I was so ready. I had already mapped out a 90 Day Plan so my next 30 days were planned out and I jumped straight in. At the end of those 30 days, I jumped straight into the next 30 days too.

I will tell you more about the bigger plan later, but the big thing for me at the end of my first 30 days was that I was on a roll. I had finally broken through the barriers that had stopped me before.

Over the whole 90 days I was able to expand my training and start running again in some of my sessions. I also started adding short sprint sessions and then some simple full body circuits. The sprints and circuits were quite modest to start with but steadily built in intensity over the whole 90 days.

By the end of 90 days, I saw some dramatic results:

- I lost over 17 and a half pounds or 8kg in bodyweight
- More importantly I also lost over 3 and a half inches from my waist.

And I wasn't just moving again, I had built regular exercise back into my life.

In fact it went so well that by March 2014 I passed the fitness test to move into basic training as a Firefighter with my local Fire & Rescue Service.

I was now making rapid progress. I went on to basic training and was fit enough to qualify as an operational Firefighter just a few weeks after my 56th birthday. See Fig 3 over the page.

What's more, I was fit enough to complete 6 years of active service into my 60s.

And in that time, I covered a whole range of incidents from House Fires to Field and Woodland Fires, from Road Collisions to Rail Incidents and a number of different animal rescues including of all things a Parrot stuck in a tree.

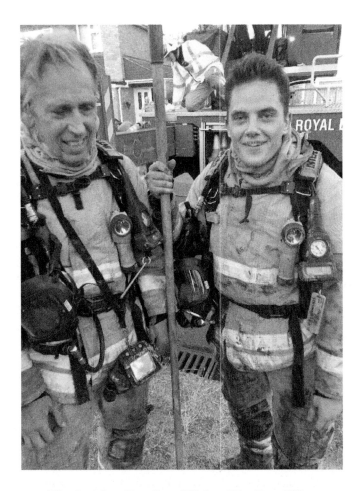

**Fig 3. After Dealing With a Big Roof Fire
(I'm on the left)**

Of course, as a Firefighter one part of you wants to be involved in a big incident, but the other part of you just wants to make sure everyone is safe and that you get the job done as quickly as possible.

I thoroughly enjoyed my years in the service and enjoyed keeping myself "Firefighter fit".

I had reclaimed my health & fitness, but it didn't stop there.

I got back in the gym to do some heavy lifting again and I got back in a rowing eight again competing in the Vets Head. I took up Obstacle Course Racing, or OCR, and even tried indoor climbing which I had always wanted to do.

But best of all I went hiking in the mountains with my kids.

## 3.4 But What About Your First 30 Days?

Using *The Power of Walking* for those first 30 days laid the foundation for me. But what if you are reading this and thinking:

- You're not sure if you can walk briskly and continuously for 20-25 mins.
- You have never exercised or trained to your metabolic levels before, how does that work?
- Scientific or not, is walking even a serious exercise?

Well that's the thing. It wasn't until I helped a couple of colleagues who wanted to train for the Fire Service that I realised that breaking through in the first 30 days was a very personal thing.

We all must start at our own level so I had to help them:

- Find a time/distance they could walk for
- Show them how to measure and maintain their metabolic level.

So, I set about creating a more detailed 30 Day Plan to help them do just that. And one that just about anyone can use to get moving again.

But I also had to explain that they couldn't expect to reclaim all their health & fitness in those 30 days. It was important to define and set expectations at a realistic level.

Yes, it's obvious and we did joke about it. But the truth is, in my own earlier attempts I failed to heed this sensible advice myself.

It all comes back to accepting where we are and starting from there.

I struggled with that, and I was just trying to help both them and you avoid the same mistake.

There was a broader aim as well, and that was to find a pattern of exercise that was:

- Doable, not something that was likely to cause strains or injuries.
- Invigorating rather than exhausting, you're training to live, not living to train.
- Fun, you should look forward to it, not feel you need some sort of iron discipline to make it happen.

I suggested that if they could find such a pattern in those first 30 days, as I had done, then they will find all sorts of ways of fitting exercise into their lifestyles well into the future.

And I'm not talking about just walking here. They might progress to running, cycling, swimming, rowing, weight training, whatever. In fact, they could end up in a completely unexpected place on their own journeys, just as I have done.

They stuck with it and by day 30 they were good and ready for the next 30 days and the same happened for the 30 after that. They both went on to qualify as Firefighters.

One of them, Harry, recently contacted me to say that even whilst working and travelling in New Zealand, he still kept to a regular training regime doing whatever exercise he could find.

Why? Because staying fit and healthy just made him feel better both physically and mentally. It seems that regular exercise is now part of his "DNA".

So, this book is dedicated to those first 30 days and is written for anyone who is looking to find a way to get active again or even for the first time. It is safe and manageable. If you can walk, you can do this.

And yet I know you might still be sceptical that this can work.

You might even try a few walks and feel like you are not really making progress at first, I get it.

But if you are going through the same loops I was caught in back in 2013 then all I can say is "Just Try It". Give it a go "For 30 days".

Set those times aside as your time and most importantly follow the instructions laid out in the plan.

You are designed to move so just go for it and let the magic happen.

.

# 4. ALL THE HURDLES GETTING IN THE WAY OF PROGRESS

Now look, I understand that you want to get active but there are some hurdles to overcome. This may be your first time exercising or you may be coming back after a long break. Either way you need to find an exercise plan that you can manage right now and one that can help you progress.

From what I have seen there are 4 big issues to address if you want to make a start from where you are physically right now, to comfortably adapt it to your lifestyle and then make it stick.

## 4.1. The Link Between Failing Fitness and Failing Health

Even now it makes me shudder when I remember how close I came to letting my health slip away for good. I just didn't understand what was happening, but I was just slowing down.

Perhaps you have noticed your energy levels, your physical, mental and emotional levels, starting to fade away. But like me, you're too young to be feeling old, surely.

Maybe you've fallen into the same trap. You monitor your weight. You might be significantly overweight and know only too well that you have a problem. Or maybe you're just a bit overweight and not overly worried about your health.

Your BMI Score could even still be hovering in the "healthy" category, I mean mine was.

Either way, that increase around the waist just creeps up and up almost unnoticed. And conversely the resulting decline of your health and fitness creeps down and down almost unnoticed too. Those imperceptible trends will continue unless you do something about them.

But there is a simple truth about human physiology:

## We are all designed to move

So, if you can get moving again then you can start to reclaim both your fitness and your health.

## 4.2. I Tried and Failed to Get Moving So Many Times

Have you tried to get active again and wondered why it didn't work?

Of course, we can all appreciate that life can get in the way and there are all sorts of things that can take up most of our time. Family commitments and work commitments are necessities of course. All these distractions make it difficult to find the time to look after yourself. But that link between your fitness and health illustrates that it is important to find a way past this.

The link between your fitness and health also highlights something that is easily overlooked. You see that slow creep of a more sedentary lifestyle comes with a twist because there is a universal truth about your physiology and your muscles and that is you must:

## Use them or lose them

And that doesn't just mean the obvious muscles like the biceps in your upper arm. No, this means all the deep muscles holding your spine in shape, the small stabiliser muscles that enable complicated joints like your shoulders to work and the muscles that pump your heart and keep your cardiovascular system pumping the blood around your body.

It doesn't matter if this is your first time exercising or if you are trying to pick up your fitness from where you left it years ago, you are in the same situation. Your muscles, the ligaments and tendons, in fact your whole body has settled into a condition suited to a sedentary lifestyle.

If you are starting exercise for the first time the challenge can seem daunting.

If you are starting again after a long break and trying to overcome this pattern of failed exercise startups you need to find a way to accept where you are, it is not a measure of you. It is what it is.

So, it doesn't matter how you have arrived at this point, your new exercise activity needs to be:

- Flexible enough to fit into your life and
- At a level of exertion you can actually manage

And it should also be enjoyable.

## 4.3 Is Walking Enough?

I remember only too clearly that sinking feeling when I finally admitted to myself that the only exercise I could manage was a brisk walk.

Maybe you've had that same feeling. I mean how is walking going to help you get back to those heady days when you could run effortlessly, or power through an erg session, let alone lift those heavy weights again? Or if this is your first time, maybe you are wondering if walking is even really an "exercise"?

You might see someone of a similar age running in the park with a strong, elegant style or another heading to the gym looking like an athlete who has just aged a bit. It may be hard to see how walking a few times a week is ever going to help you bridge that gap.

However, you must also remember this is your starting point not your end point.

Right now, you just need to get walking.

Besides, if you are already moving around during the day, then you're already walking. All we are doing is taking that natural physical movement to another level.

And once you learn a few little tweaks you'll quickly discover *The Power of Walking* for yourself. And you will discover that even "Just walking" you really can train like an athlete.

## 4.4 Losing Your Life

As you look around the different areas of your life you may be starting to see how declining health & fitness doesn't just affect you. It affects so many people around you too.

As your energy levels drop, even little by little over time, have you found yourself doing less and less with family and friends? Perhaps you have even found yourself becoming detached from close friends and family members. If you are slowly drifting apart, before you know it that gap becomes a chasm.

There were things I wanted to do with my own children before they headed off to University and the big wide world. But we had drifted apart and things just fizzled out. That left me feeling empty and crushed. I had to change to reconnect with my children before it was too late.

If you feel like you are drifting away from family and friends, you need to know that it's up to you to change. It's up to you to become the person you want to be. And when you start that journey back to being the real you, that's when you will start reconnecting.

.

# 5. OVERVIEW OF THE 30 DAY PLAN

*The Power of Walking* is all about starting your journey to reclaim your health & fitness. Getting started can be so hard, but there is a way that just about anyone can use to make it work.

Of course, this isn't going to turn your health and fitness completely around in 30 days. But this short book can change your direction of travel right around.

Instead of being stuck on a path of steady decline, even if it is almost imperceptible, you can change direction and start to grow again.

And as you change direction you will discover that your health and fitness aren't some sort of luxury extra in your life, they are foundations for a richer, fuller life.

This short book will show how you can start training like an athlete just by walking and it does this by taking you through a series of easy steps. They are so surprisingly easy that just about anybody can follow them. And yet they are also really powerful.

You can do this from home, there are no recurring fees and there are no equipment costs either. Well except maybe the purchase of a pair of shoes or trainers you find comfortable to walk in.

And 30 days in your gains will be like a springboard giving you a newfound confidence to take positive decisions and take action on the next steps of your journey. You're headed in a new direction and you're on your way back.

You have taken the first steps on your journey to reclaim your health & fitness and now you can start to grab your life back too.

# 6. THERE'S A LOT TO DO IN THE 30 DAY PLAN

Now we can start to tackle the 4 big issues. I presented them sequentially in the previous chapter and I'll do the same again here. But they are intertwined, and they impact on each other, so don't worry if you seem to be skipping from one to another, just go with the flow you are comfortable with.

## 6.1 Tackling The Impact of Failing Health

This section is about understanding the connection between your health and your fitness. More importantly, it shows you how you can make the decision to change and take accountability for your fitness and your health. It's a tough decision to carry through, but it is your decision, nonetheless.

Let me tell you right away that it is very liberating to take accountability for your own health. This simple decision changes the way you look at the whole situation, it changes your focus. Instead of worrying about what is going wrong or what you can't do, you start to focus on "What you are going to do next".

I urge you to start monitoring your Waist to Height Ratio. It's simple enough, just measure your waist and your height then divide your waist measure by your height. See Fig 4 on the following page.

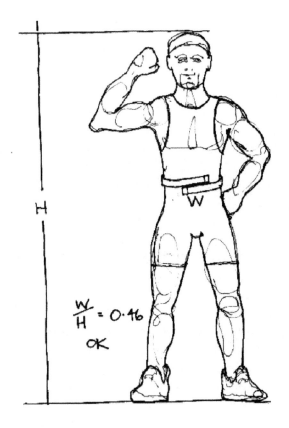

**Fig 4. Your Waist to Height Ratio**

The measure of 0.5 is a universal indicator for all adults **(Online Source 1)**. It applies regardless of your gender or your overall body type, your somatotype. A Ratio above or >0.5 indicates increasing risk of a range of horrible diseases like High Blood Pressure and Heart Attack. A Ratio below or <0.5 indicates decreasing risks of the same diseases.

Don't take my word for it, you can check out what Elizabeth Blackburn & Elissa Epel have to say on **Page** 210 of their excellent book The Telomere Effect **(Ref 1)**.

> "Subcutaneous fat, found under the skin and in the limbs, carries fewer health risks. High intra-abdominal fat is metabolically troublesome and indicates some level of poor glucose control or insulin resistance. In one study, greater WHR predicts 40 percent greater risk for telomere shortening over the next five years."

Now that you have a reliable health indicator you can decide if you really want to take action to improve your health. And one of the best things we can all do for our health is to get physically active and stay physically active. We are all designed to move and yet so many aspects of modern life steer us towards a more sedentary lifestyle.

Of course, it is hard to break free of the patterns of modern life, but we can all learn to value a more active life and the health benefits that flow from physical activity. And to do this we can take the following three steps:

1. Start to value yourself. You matter. Your fitness matters. Your health matters. It is a choice to take action to improve your health and fitness. Start today.

2. Commit to setting aside time every week dedicated to you, time when you look after your health, starting with 3 hours a week.
3. Commit to building an exercise routine that can fit in with everything else in your life.

Now that you have decided to look after your own health again, we can start.

## 6.2. Starting Out and Getting Past The False Starts

This section is all about how to crash through the initial barriers that may have stopped you in the past.

It is about setting immediate goals that are in line with your current levels of health and fitness and your current lifestyle.

It doesn't matter if this is the first time you have ever exercised or if you are coming back to exercise again after a long break. Either way, getting started can be tough.

Of course, time constraints and the pressures of modern life are factors. But there are also physical factors that often seem to be overlooked.

Maybe you have tried to get active again, and like me, you tried numerous times and different approaches. But each time you just found yourself grinding to a halt.

In my case I thought I could just "flick a switch" and regain most of the fitness of my youth.

Who was I kidding?

It required a considerable mind shift for me to let go of the past and just accept where I was in the present. But when I did finally manage to do just that, then everything changed for me.

So, I must repeat this, it doesn't matter if this is the first time you have ever exercised or if you are coming back after a long break, you still need to make one more mind shift today:

## You have to accept where you are, right now

I know this can be really difficult. If you were fit some years back It is possible that you don't want to admit how far you have fallen.

Or if this is your first time you might be struggling to see how you can ever change. You can put any such concerns to one side because you are going to start with an exercise you can manage and one you were born to do, Walking.

Let us take a moment to consider some of the immediate and obvious benefits of walking:

## The Benefits of Walking:

- Well, just about everyone can walk, it is a natural movement for us.
- Walking uses a lot of muscles besides the legs.
- Walking stimulates the cardiovascular and respiratory systems.
- Walking is relatively gentle on your muscles and gentle on your joints, particularly your hip and knee joints.
- We can all start walking at a pace or intensity that is both safe and manageable.
- We can change the intensity of the walking exercise with a few easy tweaks making it a very versatile and effective type of exercise.

In the previous section you committed to set aside three hours every week for your health and now we can start planning how we use that time.

## Now you can take action:

1. Mark three one hour slots in your diary each week.
2. Dedicate 20-25 mins to your walking exercise.
3. Now the hour slots make a bit more sense. You need a bit of time.

**Mark three one-hour slots in your diary each week.** Do this every week and dedicate these to your health. Ideally make two of these in the normal week and one at the weekend. Over the next few weeks, you might find yourself juggling these around to find a more comfortable fit with your overall lifestyle and that is just fine. If it helps, you can download a simple weekly planner (see Page 49). The key is to mark and highlight these three one-hour slots prominently in your diary. These are three hours of "You Time".

**Dedicate 20-25 mins to your walking exercise.** And do this in each of the one hour slots. So right at the start you need to explore your area to find some locations or routes where you will enjoy walking continuously for your 20-25 minutes exercise in each one hour slot. I appreciate that these areas must be places where you feel comfortable and safe. This is also about getting out in the fresh air so you can enjoy whatever the weather is doing and watch the birds or other wildlife, or even other people.

**Treat the whole one-hour slots as "You Time".** Now the one-hour slots make a bit more sense. You need a bit of time to get ready, maybe a few minutes to make your way to your walking route loosening up along the way, then a few minutes to get back and finally getting back to your regular day. These little bits of time are also part of each of the one-hour time slots and they are part of "You Time". Enjoy the anticipation of the walking, the satisfaction of finishing your walk and how much better you feel. If you still have a few minutes left, then start planning something you really want to do with your family or friends.

Over the next few weeks, you might find yourself juggling these around to find a more comfortable fit with your overall lifestyle and that is just fine.

## A few caveats:

**What if 20-25 mins walking is too much?** That's fine, just find what you can manage and start there. This is your plan, find what you can comfortably manage and go from there.

**Can't do 3 slots a week?** Look I get it, you might have young children or be looking after a relative, or be overloaded with work, I've been there. So, try to make sure you do 2 to start with. And as you progress just try to find when you can start doing the third.

**Can't do anything during the regular working week?** That's fine, just do 2 on the weekend. And again, as you progress just try to find ways to fit a third in during your regular week if you can.

Look, the point here is to find ways to just get started in a way that fits easily into your current lifestyle. As you get underway you will find that you will start to explore ways to make it work because you have committed to take accountability for your health. It just sort of happens.

## 6.3. Can You Train Like an Athlete by Walking?

This section gets to the very heart of this simple but effective plan. I might feel inclined to say "Trust Me" on this because it works.

But I think it is much more appropriate to explain the science behind it and then suggest that you try it for yourself. But I mean genuinely try it out.

And it's OK, I'll understand if you are still sceptical and you are asking yourself how walking can work? Is it really possible to train like an athlete by walking?

The secret is to use a method called Heart-rated Training. With this method it is not a matter of how fast you are going or if you are even walking or running.

We are going back to the basic principles of Heart-rated Training developed by Prof Laurence E. Morehouse who helped create the fitness programme for the astronauts destined for the first lunar landings.

Prof Morehouse and his team at UCLA identified that the individual astronauts in their care responded best by training to their individual metabolic bands.

Now others working in this field made similar observations. But Prof Morehouse identified that this same principle worked for less athletic people, like himself.

He went on to write a fitness book Total Fitness in 30 Minutes a Week, co-authored by Leonard Gross (**Ref 2**) for people like himself.

And in this book, he explains that the reason why Heart-rated Exercise works is this:

**It is not how fast you go
that improves your fitness,
it is the metabolic effect you create.**

So you don't have to run as fast as an Olympic Athlete to improve your fitness, you just have to train in a way that creates the same metabolic effect.

This means we can all use the same concepts of Training Bands and Heart-rated Training just as effectively as any elite athlete.

You might be thinking that the science has moved on since 1977 and of course it has.

But now things get really exciting because more recent research backs up the underlying principles of Heart-rated Training and provides an easier way to identify our individual training bands.

So more recent research identifies a training zone you will be able to achieve that is really effective in boosting your fitness. This is the Z1 Training Zone shown in Fig 5 below. Some sources claim that you can achieve up to 90% of your fitness potential by training in this

Z1 Zone. We can debate the exact figure another time. But what is certainly true is that this Training Zone is effective for everyone.

And please be aware that there are any number of classifications of these bands or zones. But we can use three shown in Fig 5 for the moment. If, or rather when you progress you might also use other classifications which is fine because that is all part of your progression.

| Zone or Band | Description | Lactate/hr points |
|---|---|---|
| **Z1** | Extensive endurance compensation training | Lactate level below 2mmol/L, heart rate less than 80% of maximum "low lactate base training" |
| **Z2** | Intensive endurance | Lactate 2-4 mmol/L 80-85% HRmax **"no man's land"** |
| **Z3** | High-intensity endurance Race specific velocity-endurance | Lactate >4mmoll/L Above threshold Velocity training to induce lactate accumulation, ie "high intensity intervals" |

**Fig 5. Training Zones**

From Advanced Fitness Training for elite sports performance (Editor Andrew Hamilton 2010). **(Ref 3)** With the kind permission of the publishers.

BUT for this to work you need to approach this as though you are a serious athlete:

- You will train, or rather walk at a fast pace so that your muscles are creating lactate, but the pace is just fast enough that your muscles are also utilising the lactate and not allowing it to accumulate.
- We could undergo a detailed assessment to find what your personal heart rate would be in this ideal "Zone" and use a heart rate monitor to keep you in the "Zone" as you walk. But there is a simpler way.
- We will use a universal measure called the "Talk Test" described below.

The parameters we need to observe in order to effectively use the "Talk Test" are as follows:

- If you are walking at a pace and can still comfortably hold a conversation, then I am sorry but that is NOT fast enough.
- If you are walking at a pace a but can barely say a short sentence, then you are walking TOO fast.
- If you are walking at a pace and can say a moderately long sentence but can't engage in comfortable conversation, then you are JUST ABOUT RIGHT.

The origin and application of the "Talk Test" is described by Pavel Tsatsouline in his book, Kettlebell Simple and Sinister **(Ref 4)**.

If we go back to **Fig 5**, then we can start to see that the "Talk Test" is demonstrating how hard your respiratory system is working.

As you walk faster and you start working harder, the production of Lactate increases. This requires more and more oxygen to process it and so your breathing becomes a little harder.

But if you go too fast, even though your breathing becomes much harder the body cannot break down the lactate quickly enough and it starts to accumulate. That is when you move into the Z2 Zone and breathing becomes noticeably hard.

But we don't need to go there in this 30-day plan. We can stay in Z1 and take advantage of the fact that everyone can build a very significant level of fitness by training effectively at this Z1 level.

The simple but effective "Talk Test" means that we can all experiment and find the pace where we can stay in the Z1 Zone. And if you're interested, the moderately long sentence I used for my "Talk Test" was and still is:

## "Am I going Fast Enough?"

The second indicator of your Z1 Zone is that it shouldn't exhaust you. Even at the end of 20-25 mins you should feel tired but not exhausted. It should feel like you can quite happily continue for another 5-10 mins. And after winding down and just a short rest, you should feel good to go for the rest of your day.

Even so, starting out this Z1 can feel quite hard going for some.

But remember, you are not walking yourself into exhaustion, you are simply walking to create the right metabolic effect. In fact, it won't take many weeks before you will find that you can keep that pace for 10's of minutes without being unduly tired at the end.

BUT in order for this to work you **MUST** make sure that in each of your 3 sessions you do **Walk at a Z1 Pace for the full 20-25 mins**.

So, if you are walking with a friend, you can say the odd sentence to each other, but if you are having a chat, then I am sorry, but you are not going fast enough.

Remember you are training like an athlete for these 20-25 mins, you can have your chat when you have finished.

And don't get distracted. If you bump into a friend just say, "Hi and Bye, I'm Training" and finish your 20-25 mins. This is your time. This is time dedicated to your health. Any good friend will respect that.

## Terminology

There is a lot of confusion around terminology. Some people might try and describe the exercise described above as Cardio, others might call it CV or Steady State and others still might call it UT2. There are nuances which we can cover another time.

For the moment can I suggest that we put those terms to one side and simply refer to this as Z1 Training in line with the data shown in **Fig 5**.

## Walking Tips

There is a huge range of material online offering advice on walking covering topics like stride length, foot placement and so forth. I urge you to become a student and explore the resources out there. On my own journey I did find three tips particularly useful:

1. Posture
2. Hands
3. Swinging your arms as you walk

But these are not widely covered. So, I will cover them here as follows:

**Posture -** Of course we want to encourage you to walk with a good upright posture. I came across a solution that works for me quite by accident many years ago.

It's an essential element of The Alexander Technique and it requires you to try to lift your (whole) head as you walk. Your head needs to be balanced in a neutral position of course and I found the chin is a really useful guide in that respect. My original source was a book by Sarah Barker called, The Alexander Technique, The revolutionary way to use your body for total energy **(Ref 5 & Online Source 3)**, published back in 1978.

I am not an expert in this field and there are more up to date books available. So, I have included a useful online source in the references at the end of the book should you wish to find out more about this particular technique.

I was also lucky enough to spend some time with an "old school" rowing coach. He coached junior girls with considerable success and his crews were always identifiable by their excellent posture and technique.

He would encourage the girls to imagine that somebody was lifting them by their hair as they rowed/sculled.

I tried the same with a group I was coaching.

Now it has to be said that some responded well but others ignored it. But that is an important point because just like the girls in the rowing squad, you need to find what works for you. But what I can say is that if you can lift your head as you walk it is like a release allowing you to walk more freely.

**Hands, or rather your Thumbs -** Notice how your hands hang by your side as you stand still. If the thumbs are turned inwards, then try turning them to point forwards and then outwards. Can you feel your shoulders opening and turning back a little. If so, you are gently unpicking that unhealthy forward shoulder roll many of us accumulate from sitting, driving and various other modern reasons for poor posture.

**Swinging your Arms as You Walk -** From now on, as you walk make sure your hands are free. Let your hands and arms swing in their natural motion. And notice your thumbs. Try keeping them pointed forwards (see **Hands** above) as they swing by your hips.

I know, you may feel a bit self-conscious at first, it might feel like you are "marching". But honestly, who is going to notice. Let them swing and enjoy how good that natural movement feels. Oh, by the way, hopefully you will have worked out that trying to walk at Z1 holding a cup of coffee is a No No!

There is a lot to take in in this section, but THE REALLY BIG POINT is to experiment to find your genuine Z1 pace and then walk at your Z1 Pace for your 3 sessions of 20-25 mins. I can only encourage you to trust the science. Go with it and explore how you really can train like an athlete. This has to be the most exciting part of this book.

Then just try each of the different tweaks one at a time over the 30 days and test out the effects for yourself. If they work for you just let the small adjustments become easy habits.

## 6.4. Getting Your Life Back

This section is all about the bigger picture. Of course, I had always thought that my health and my fitness were important to me. But back in the bad days before I found the way to turn things around, I had lost sight of this. I had lost sight of the basic truth that my health and fitness were actually key foundations for my whole life. They were not just added extras.

As my health and fitness both fell into decline my whole life fell into decline and I was drifting away from family and friends. This drift was almost imperceptible until it came into sharp relief with my kids.

In my own teens some close family friends introduced me to hiking the mountains. Those trips made a huge impression on me and as a result I developed a love of the great outdoors. There was one particular area of the mountains that became "my special place".

When my own kids were heading off to University and the big wide world, I didn't have the energy or capacity to do for them what others had done for me.

Through their growing years I had wanted to share that special place with them. They might or might not take to it the same way I had, but I wanted to let them at least share it and then let them each decide as they may. I felt that I had really let them down.

But I decided that whilst my effort might be late, it wasn't too late to try again.

So, as I started my journey back, I told them about my own experiences back in my teens. I told them about my special place and how I would like to take them there so that they could explore the mountains in the way I was able to.

And I told them I was getting myself ready to do that, but it would take me a little while yet.

I left it with them to decide if they wanted to take me up on the offer.

It didn't happen straight away; I had a lot of ground to make up. In fact, it took close to 18 months.

But they watched me getting myself back into shape again. They saw the maps I bought and the new compass. Without realising it we started planning it together.

And it did happen. We got there. Hiking those mountains seemed to heal all those years of drifting apart. I had my family back.

So, look, the important message in this section is that your health and fitness are the foundations of your life.

If there is something you need or want to do with your family or friends, then don't wait for some moment in the future when you think you are going to be ready.

Get started straight away, even if it is simply planning what you would like to do in a few months.

Start right now. Explore the things you want to share with your family, friends and loved ones. Let the connections grow again. It might be slow at first, but you will start to grow stronger every week now.

And you know what? People will see you getting stronger again. They will feel it. They will want to be part of it.

You really can get your life back in so many ways.

# 7. READ THIS BEFORE YOU START

It does not matter if you were super fit back in the day or if this is the first time you have ever tried to build any sort of fitness into your life. Either way you need to understand why we are starting out just walking.

You are quite literally rebooting your whole body. Moving from a sedentary lifestyle to an active lifestyle you just need to let everything ease back into life. And everything includes:

- Your big muscles like your quads and calves
- Your Cardiovascular system and your heart
- Your Respiratory system and your lungs
- The Core and Ab muscles that give you a healthy spine.
- The Stabiliser muscles that enable complex joints like your shoulders and knees to work effectively.
- The fascia around the muscles that should stretch, and glide freely but probably needs a bit of releasing.
- The joint capsules that need to loosen up and reactivate their magical synovial fluids that lubricate and nourish your joints.
- All the ligaments that hold the joints together that need to be teased back into life.
- All the tendons that hold the muscles in place that also need to be teased back into life.

There are probably other aspects of your physiology that we should mention here, but this list makes the point. There will be a lot going on as you ease your body back into an active lifestyle.

But that's absolutely fine because walking should allow us all to start rebooting these aspects of our fitness without any real risk of injury or strain. And walking fast enough to operate in our genuine Z1 Zone will speed up that process because of the metabolic effect created.

Before I developed my walking plan, I tried several other methods. But each time I disregarded, or more accurately I ignored that list. Of course, I failed miserably each time. I put my back out, I aggravated an old knee injury and triggered a number of other unwanted outcomes.

It was only when I heeded the advice that I gave to the juniors that I started to make real progress. And I repeat that advice again here:

### Accept where you are, train to your metabolic levels and then let the magic happen.

You see "the magic" is not just the fitness returning to your big muscles and your cardiovascular system, it is all the other aspects starting to ease back into life.

.

# 8. THE 30 DAY PLAN

I know you are keen to get straight into it, but there are a few things you need to do in order to be ready to start. You need to plan your routes and take your measurements.

## Planning your Routes

Have a look around your neighbourhood and find an area or areas where you will enjoy walking and where you feel safe, especially for you ladies.

You might have to travel a short distance; I mean I have a 5-10 minute walk to my different start points.

Remember we are trying to do everything in one hour if possible, but if you have to travel a bit, say to a park or river side walk or a country lane then just factor this into your time.

Now test out possible routes and just see how far you can walk in 20 to 25 minutes. This can be a circular route or walking 10 to 12 and a half minutes out and back.

Remember we are aiming for a walk of 20-25 mins at your Z1 pace.

Let's say you are doing this from home. Try out each element so that you can estimate of how long the whole session will take you. The elements include:

- Stop everything and get ready.
- Leave home and make your way to your start point.
- Complete your walk.
- Return home.
- Get ready to resume your day.

Now you can see why I suggested setting aside an hour for each of your walking sessions.

## Taking Your Measurements and Recording Progress

And now there are three more things to do:

1. Take and record your measurements.
2. Calculate your Waist to Height Ratio
3. Start recording your progress

You can download two useful charts here:

(https://www.dropbox.com/s/6fk5ou294ikmfti/Measurement%20and%20Planning%20Charts.doc?dl=1)

The download includes:

- Measurement Charts
- Weekly Planner

There are two different Measurement Charts, so you can use either to suit.

Now in order to calculate your Waist to Height Ratio you do need to accurately measure your waist.

So as to avoid any confusion I suggest using the method approved by The World Cancer Research Fund (**Online Source 2**) and illustrated in Fig 6 below.

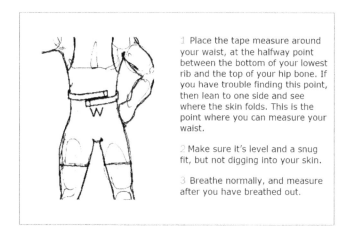

1 Place the tape measure around your waist, at the halfway point between the bottom of your lowest rib and the top of your hip bone. If you have trouble finding this point, then lean to one side and see where the skin folds. This is the point where you can measure your waist.

2 Make sure it's level and a snug fit, but not digging into your skin.

3 Breathe normally, and measure after you have breathed out.

### Fig 6. How to Accurately Measure Your Waist

This might come as a bit of a surprise, especially if you have more subcutaneous fat sitting around the waist and a little below this measuring level.

But as we noted back on Page 31, it is the deeper fat, the visceral fat lying within the abdomen, that is of particular concern regarding our health.

As a quick reminder I repeat Fig 4 from Page 30 as Fig 7 below. This shows you how to then measure your Waist to Height Ratio.

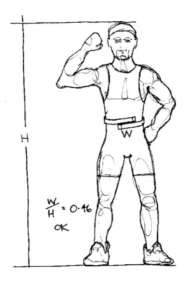

$$\frac{W}{H} = 0.46$$
OK

**Fig 7. Your Waist to Height Ratio**

And also included in the download is a simple Weekly Planner.

Now this might seem a little too enthusiastic. But actually I found it really useful to plan out each week and then jot down any notes. These may have been about how I found the walking, or possible changes to my routes, or just interesting observations.

I still have these and years later they make interesting reading. So, the Weekly Planner is there if you want to use it.

You might not be too pleased to hear this, but I would also suggest taking a photo or two to show the shape you are in as you start this Plan. I regret not doing that.

But luckily a friend of mine "Alan the Artist" captured my sorry state, so I will share that with you to encourage you to take the photos. See Fig 8 below:

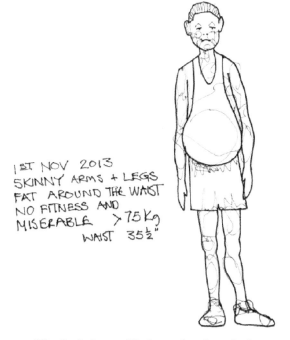

1ST NOV 2013
SKINNY ARMS + LEGS
FAT AROUND THE WAIST
NO FITNESS AND
MISERABLE  > 75Kg
WAIST 35½"

**Fig 8. A Sorry Sight – the dreaded Middle-Age Spread**

PS. I was so embarrassed by my bulging waistline that I couldn't even write down the true figure. It was well over 37 inches.

But don't despair. You are just starting out so it's important to remember where you are headed.

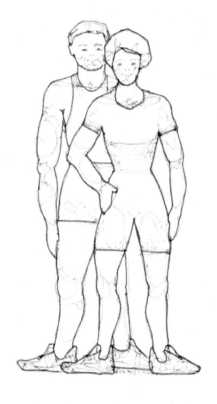

**Fig 9. You Can Do This**

**So, let's get started**

## Days 0-7

Start by selecting three one-hour time slots and then mark them on your Weekly Planner or in your diary, whichever you have chosen to use.

Ideally, I suggest trying to do these in the regular working week so that you keep weekends free for social activities.

But I understand that this can be difficult so maybe use one weekend day. And look, if that is too difficult then don't fret about it and just use both weekend days.

And honestly, if two sessions on the weekend are all you can manage right now, just run with it. After all, I explain in Chapter 9 how I could only exercise on the weekends for a while.

The important thing is to get started. And now that you are walking you can make a point to use these sessions to experiment with the "Talk Test". Adjust your pace, get a handle on what you can comfortably manage and still enjoy doing.

Remember you are training like an athlete now. Your pace is important, and we want to get it right so that you are training in your genuine Z1 Zone.

And the last thing to do is record the time/distance of your walks. That is easy to do if you have one of these fitness trackers.

But don't worry if you haven't. Just note your start and finish positions and then time your walks so you can compare times from session to session and week to week.

I should point out that you are not in a hurry here. Concentrate on your genuine Z1 pace and let the magic happen.

And I also suggest using the Weekly Planners to record any notes and store these in a file for future reference.

## Days 8-14

Now you can adjust your three one-hour time slots if you need to in order to make them easier to fit into your regular daily activities. Get on and do them and record everything in the Weekly Planner.

When you are completing your main 20-25 min walking session, use the "Talk Test" regularly so that you get used to monitoring and holding your pace in your Z1 Zone. It does take a little while to get used to this.

Remember, if you are walking with a friend and you can chat freely then you are not walking fast enough.

And if you happen to bump into someone you know, just say "Hi and Bye. I am training" and finish your walk. Actually, your walk is now a "Z1 Training Session".

And as you do all this you can refer back to Chapter 6 Section 3 and start experimenting with:

- Your chin position and your posture
- Your hand/thumb position and arm swings.

When you record your times and distances for the week you can also jot down any notes on how you felt at the end of each session. And record any interesting observations along the way, even if there has been any change in your sleep.

## Days 15-21

Once again you start the week by making any adjustments to your three one-hour time slots to make sure that they fit really easily into your week.

You're getting the hang of this now, so you know it's important to make sure you are staying in your Z1 Zone using:

- The Talk Test

You're now going to start assessing how well you walk, in other words your "Form" by monitoring your:

- Chin position to hold a strong posture.
- Hand/Thumb positions and flowing arm swings

And you finish the week by recording your times and distances and noting any interesting observations, how you feel, interesting sights and how you are sleeping.

## Days 22-28

Your time slots are working well, you are holding your Z1 pace easily and your "Form" is developing nicely.

So, this week you can start to experiment and test yourself.

- Can you walk a little faster and still meet the "Talk Test"?
- Or can you now walk a bit further without feeling overly tired?
- Are you feeling more cheerful walking tall with your chin held a little higher?
- Do you feel like your arm swings are flowing smoothly as you walk?
- Do your shoulders feel a little more open and loose because of your hand position?

Now before your week is over, I strongly urge you to:

1. Record your times and distances for the week.
2. Use the prompts above to make a note of any interesting observations.

But you're not done yet.

Using your downloaded charts, you now need to:

1. Take, record and compare your new measurements.
2. Calculate and compare your new Waist to Height Ratio

And add these details to your weekly records. Your file of Weekly Planners will provide a great record of your progress so file them away safely.

## Day 28 - More To Do

Part of starting to value your health and fitness, your time, and you, is to start celebrating your wins and gains.

You have made it to Day 28. You got moving and now you are active again. You have just broken through some really tough hurdles and barriers.

And what have your measurements revealed? Has anything changed? You might have lost a little bit of weight, but more importantly:

## Has your waist measurement changed?

But that's not the only measurement, is it? Have you extended your walks? Are you walking a little faster? Or do you just feel better as you walk?

Any and all of these little gains are worth celebrating because they represent a change in your direction of travel.

And now the big question, are you feeling ready to start consolidating those gains and step up a level? Not a huge step, just a big enough step to keep making progress.

You'll know if you are ready.

## Days 29-30

If you are feeling ready to move on then you can check your options such as a more vigorous programme to continue your journey.

If you want to continue developing your fitness through walking you can always check out the full "Walk, Run, Train Plan" I used as the foundation to get "Firefighter fit".

Or you might have other plans like joining a walking or running group, or a gym or fitness class.

The important thing is to transition to the next activity or programme straight away and take advantage of the momentum you have built up over the last 28 days.

And remember, you might move on to another activity or programme, but keep checking to make sure you can fit it into your lifestyle and that you are enjoying it.

You can always adjust or even switch around to make sure you find it easy to stick with it.

## Days 29-36

But what if you just don't feel quite ready to step up to a more challenging activity or programme yet?

That's fine, you can always repeat part or all of the 30 day plan again. You can make it more challenging to make sure that you continue rebuilding your fitness.

For example, you could:
- Extend the walks so if you walked for 20 mins, now you walk for 30 mins.
- Increase your pace, but still make sure to use the Talk Test to keep in your Z1 Zone
- Add in some hilly sections to your walk.
- Find a way to fit the 3 sessions into the regular week and make sure to include social activities on the weekends.
- Start running for part of each walk or one complete walking distance.

From my own experience and chatting to a few of the people I have helped already, you will know when you are good and ready to move up a level.

## What Could You Do Next?

Back in Nov 2013 I submitted my application to join the Fire & Rescue Service in the same week that I started my journey.

I was serious in that I was going to give it my best shot, but I really had no idea if I could turn my health and fitness around enough to actually make it.

I was genuinely surprised how much progress I made in the first 30 days. And that success was a real springboard to make further progress.

I was still surprised when I passed the fitness test to progress to basic training. And to be honest the recruiting officer was probably more surprised than I was.

That was the start of a rather special six years.

What was even more surprising were all the other new opportunities that opened up.

I mean I had never even heard of Obstacle Course Racing (OCR) before and yet ended up heading off with other crew members to various events like RatRace held in early May each year.

I also got back in a Racing Eight to race the Vets Head which was a bit sobering I might add. Dang, we came second by one second.

And I finally got to try indoor climbing which was a real hoot. So much to do.

But best of all, I got to go hiking in the mountains with my kids. And for me that's just the best, because it makes you feel like you are on top of the world.

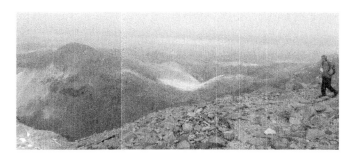

**Fig 10. Back on Top of the World**

So the big question now is:

# What can you do?

Are there any special plans you can start to make now?

If you're a bit hesitant, maybe you don't want to tempt fate, then just pencil in one or two big ones and then find a few intermediate goals that you can use as steppingstones.

And you just don't know where all this might lead you.

I mean I never really expected to be jumping off a high tower into a pool of water. 7m doesn't look so high from the bottom!

But for some strange reason I really enjoyed that jump and looked forward to it every time I returned to RatRace.

That's me on the right below in Fig 11 below.

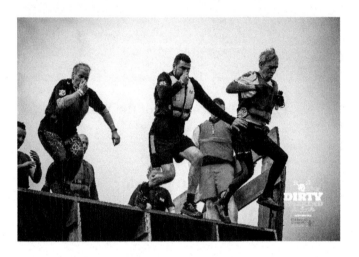

**Fig 11. The Big Water Jump at RatRace 2022**

# 9. USING THE 30 DAY – SECOND TIME AROUND

## I should have done this sooner

I mentioned earlier that I should have written this book back in 2013/2014 when I first put it into action. But I was distracted by my new role as a Firefighter. I did pass it on to a few people to help them get started and two of the lads ended up signing up as Firefighters as well.

For whatever reason I didn't write it and my notes just sat there along with all my records of workouts and training programmes as well as my research. I had moved on and enjoyed using various training protocols to develop specific strength or endurance goals. These included:

- Heavy weights, especially my favourite, the deadlift
- Kettlebells, oh how I wish I had discovered these sooner.
- Different erg and running routines for endurance and VO2 Max
- Exercises I could never do even when I was rowing competitively like proper pull ups and full body dips.

As Covid happened I wasn't too badly affected at first. I could still take the dog on long hikes, and I had an ergo plus a selection of Kettlebells to do a range of training types at home.

## Things Started to Go Wrong

But by Aug 2021 things started to go a bit wayward. Karma the dog just got a little older and didn't like trotting along at a pace for miles, so those walks just sort of fizzled out. I didn't really notice how I started to lose a bit of flexibility and mobility without them. And that was compounded because I was forced to work from home due to the Covid restrictions. My life had suddenly become more sedentary again.

There then followed a sequence of self-inflicted injuries and half-hearted recoveries as I tried to get myself ready for RatRace 2022. It was going to be the last one ever, so I couldn't miss it. 20 miles of hills, mud, some swimming and wading and 200 obstacles including the 7m water jump. I mean, what's not to love?

Despite being laid up for weeks on end twice in the period Oct 2021 to Feb 2022 I did make it to RatRace. I even got around in a reasonable time. I did miss a couple of the obstacles, but I also got over a couple of the high walls I had struggled with in earlier years. But I also injured my leg in a clumsy fall. Foolishly I did not get medical attention on the day thinking it was just (badly) bruised I could clean the cut up myself and it would be fine.

The injury didn't heal up, it got worse. I ended up at the hospital a couple of weeks later. The cut should have been stitched up on the day, oh and yes the bruising? Well there's probably a hairline fracture but it's too late to do anything about that now. And on top of all that there's now a deep infection. My wife was not happy and I got a real telling off from the nurse.

And the end result? I had to avoid putting any weight on my right leg for the next couple of months, at least, and start a course of heavy-duty antibiotics.

Just as things couldn't get any worse I then got Covid. Well one benefit of that was that it laid me out and I was bed ridden for over three weeks. This helped me keep the weight off the right leg. But then I had a reaction to the antibiotics and was covered all over with sores.

As a result, I spent most of May, June and July laid out with either the leg injury, Covid or this violent reaction to the antibiotics.

## Oh Dear, I'm Back Over 0.5

All the ups and downs of the previous 12 months and the Covid restrictions before that had an unwelcome impact.

I had become more sedentary again. I had just drifted into that state by circumstances, but this drift was especially noticeable during May, June and July, I had put on weight around the waistline again. And that was despite eating a healthy diet. It was nowhere near as bad as last time, but I did edge over the 0.5 marker.

So, my fitness had tumbled away with each delay and my health was on a downward turn as well. I was almost back to square one. It was time to get walking again.

## Back to Walking

Now before all these setbacks I had been thinking about entering a mountain marathon event in Sept of 2022. I mean that sounds fun right! But through the spring I realised this was not going to happen, so I had settled on a local Half Marathon in Oct. It's a bit unusual because it is a hilly one.

By June I realised that wasn't going to happen either. By the end of July I decided that I should at least enter the 10k event that ran parallel to the half marathon. I wanted to support my local event and I needed a goal.

But after the prolonged layoff the only exercise I could manage was a brisk walk. And even that was still a bit painful on the right shin. My wife refused to speak to me and my daughter rolled her eyes. You know, the usual family support.

## The Power of Walking

I started walking again on 1st August 2022. I was really busy with work, so I only managed two sessions a week every Saturday and Sunday. Looking on the bright side, that gave the right shin plenty of rest as it was still quite tender.

Although I couldn't run, my endurance had held up surprisingly well so I could manage 4, then 5 and then 6 miles at a good Z1 Pace. So each week I just added an extra hill and a bit more distance.

On 1st September I switched to running, again just twice a week, but over the same hilly routes. The event was in the diary now, Sunday 9th October.

Through September the right shin seemed to clear up at last and my form improved, so I was quite happy. I wasn't going to break any records, that's for sure, but I was confident I would make it up that big hill and hang on right to the finish line.

I told myself I wasn't bothered about my time, I was just going to enjoy the event.

But of course, you are surrounded by other runners and it's hard not to get a bit competitive again. So, when I saw my time I felt a bit deflated.

My daughter saw my disappointment and quickly reminded me:

### Jeepers Dad! You only started running again in September!

We both laughed, but my wife rolled her eyes. I could guess what she was thinking:

### It's not that bloomin' mountain marathon next is it?

At that point I realised that I had better do the washing up and keep a low profile for a bit.

## The Waist

Yes, that is trimming back down.

I was going to get to work on trimming my waist a bit more seriously after that 10k run. But there was another 10k in November. It's hilly and cross country which is much more enjoyable than road running. And it's in support of one of the local schools.

What can I say? The journey back to fitness and health is full of unexpected and enjoyable turns, distractions and challenges. I wouldn't have it any other way. I'll get back to the pull ups and dips over the winter, honest.

## The Mountains

With all the commotions of the last 12-15 months the next trip hiking in the mountains has been put off. But not to worry, we're on it for next year. There is a walk along Hadrian's Wall with one of my cousins and a couple of the kids might make that. But that will be an extra.

"My special place" has become "Our special place". We're heading back there soon.

# 10. FAQS

**How can I do this if I have never exercised?** If you have been walking even short distances, down the garden or to the local shop, or whatever then you already know how to do this. It's just a matter of doing a bit more in a specific way. And see the next Question.

**How can I do this if I can't walk for 20 mins?** Don't panic and don't worry about finding your Z1 just yet. Just find a distance you can walk comfortably and try to do that three times a week. It might take you a few weeks to extend that to 15 or 20 mins. Once you can do all three for at least 20 mins then start your 30 days.

**Can walking really improve fitness?** This gets to the very crux of Heart-rated Exercise. It is not your level of activity relative to anyone else that matters, it is the metabolic effect of that activity on you. To start with you might only be able to walk at a relatively slow pace and still achieve your Z1 Zone. As you progress you find yourself walking faster to achieve the same metabolic effect. Eventually you might even need to run to achieve that same effect. So yes, walking can improve your fitness if you use the Talk Test to find your genuine Z1 level.

**Will it take a long time to see any positive fitness gains?** This is a tricky question and gets to the very heart of why I wrote this short book. You might not notice much improvement in your fitness in these first 30 days. But there are subtle changes that change everything for you. You will establish a pattern of exercise back in your life, you'll learn how to make walking really effective and most importantly of all, you are moving again. Stick with it and you will enjoy one of the great benefits of Heart-rated Exercise because once you are over that initial start-up hurdle your fitness will improve surprisingly fast.

**Am I too old for this?** Look I used this in my 50s first time around and again in my 60s after a few health setbacks. If you can walk, then you can use this.

**I'm in my 20s, am I too young for this?** The only reason I didn't mention the 20s in the book is that in your 20s most people still feel a bit of that indestructibleness of youth. But two young guys asked me for help to regain their fitness. One was 19, the other 20. They had just never done any sport or serious exercise. They rebuilt their health and fitness and they both went on to become Firefighters. So yes, it still works even if you're in your 20s.

**How much is this going to cost me?** The only costs are the price of the book which is probably less than the cost of a coffee and Danish, and a pair of walking shoes/trainers if you don't already own a pair. I hope the cost is so low that it just isn't a barrier to trying this out.

**Do I need to join a gym or pay any membership?**
No. You can do all this from home or from your work if you walk during a lunch break. You can look at other options once you are moving again and feel more confident about what works for you.

# 11. YOU'VE COMPLETED THE 30 DAY PLAN, WHAT NEXT?

Right at the start I asked if you were already looking at your next challenge which may be something like:

- "10,000 Steps a Day" or "Couch to 5k"
- Joining a local walking group to go hiking.
- Joining a running group like Park Run
- Re-joining your old sports club
- Signing up at the Gym to start Weight Training again.

These are just a few ideas, but maybe you already had something else in mind. Either way I wish you every success.

But what if you still are looking for ways to build on the progress made over the last 30 days. If that is the case then you might also be interested in the full *Walk, Run, Train - 90 Day Plan* that I used to build regular exercise into my life AND as the foundation to get "Firefighter fit". Let me tell you a bit about it.

## We All Have Two Things in Common

You might recall from Chapter 4 that I highlighted a simple truth about human physiology:

**We are all designed to move.**

Well, now that you are moving again, we can expand on this point and introduce a second aspects of movement we all have in common.

## We are all designed to work at different metabolic levels.

Now we can re-visit Fig 5, from Page 39 which identifies three different metabolic levels referred to as Z1, Z2 and Z3. This is presented again in Fig 12 below.

| Zone or Band | Description | Lactate/hr points |
| --- | --- | --- |
| Z1 | Extensive endurance compensation training | Lactate level below 2mmol/L, heart rate less than 80% of maximum<br><br>"low lactate base training" |
| Z2 | Intensive endurance | Lactate 2-4 mmol/L<br><br>80-85% HRmax<br><br>**"no man's land"** |
| Z3 | High-intensity endurance Race specific velocity-endurance | Lactate >4mmol/L<br><br>Above threshold<br><br>Velocity training to induce lactate accumulation, ie<br><br>"high intensity intervals" |

### Fig 12. Training Zones Revisited

You might be surprised to find out that even walking you can still train to levels Z2 and even Z3. Yes, we can all do Z3 or "Sprints".

Back on Page 38 I highlighted the reason why Heart-rated Exercise works as follows:

**It is not how fast you go
that improves your fitness,
it is the metabolic effect you create.**

So, you don't have to run as fast as an Olympic Athlete to improve your fitness, you just have to train in a way that creates the same metabolic effect.

And even walking, you can exercise at Z2. In fact, you can even exercise at Z3. You can do the equivalent of Sprints whilst still walking!

Over the 30 days of *The Power of Walking* Plan you used the Z1 Training Zone to get moving again. Now you can move things onto another level.

## Build Regular Exercise Into Your Life with Heart-rated Training

You might be in the early stages of reclaiming your fitness, but you now have the tools to get the absolute maximum from Heart-rated Training.

And the *Walk, Run, Train* Plan shows how anyone can use the three training levels, Z1, Z2 & Z3, to rapidly build their fitness and strength. This then has a knock on effect to health as well.

Of course, this is still a simplistic introduction to the world of fitness, strength and health. But this same idea of training at different levels of exertion also works for training at different levels of strength too.

The *Walk, Run, Train* Plan introduces the next two training zones over the 90 Days.

And it shows you how to combine them in individual sessions, through the week and through each month.

The main manual covers the science behind the concept of **Heart-rated Training** so that you can get the absolute most out of the training.

It also covers some background of human physiology explaining why your shape might be a more important indicator of your health than your weight. And the Plan takes you from a walking start, to running, sprinting and full body training.

Hence the full title:

## Walk, Run Train - 90 Day Plan to build regular exercise into your life

**You can find out more at: www.walkruntrain.com**

There is some overlap with the 30 day plan presented in this book. But if you have enjoyed and benefited from the 30 day plan, then you're ready to take on the full *Walk, Run, Train - 90 Day Plan*.

By the way, you don't have to sign up with your local Fire & Rescue service though. You probably have other long term goals you're aiming for.

If you follow the link above, you might feel you can skip past the introduction because you'll be familiar with a lot of it now.

But still check out the free bonuses. These are a collection of short training videos introducing a gentle warm up routine together with essential core and upper body exercises.

If you follow the "90 Day Plan" all the way through Stages 1, 2 and 3 you will find yourself training like a real athlete. And you might also be surprised that the training leaves you invigorated rather than exhausted.

## 90 Days and Beyond

At this point you can either follow the plan through a 4th Stage, and take your training to another level again. This is the same training I used to get myself Firefighter Fit.

Or you might be feeling ready to progress to different training protocols like joining a gym again or taking up other sports like cycling or swimming.

Either way, you will be well prepared so you will find it easier than you might have ever thought possible to make regular exercise, or training, an enjoyable and unmissable part of your everyday lifestyle.

If you want to take the challenge and see where you could be in another 90 Days, then:

**Find out more at: www.walkruntrain.com**

And follow the link to:

## Walk, Run Train - 90 Day Plan to build regular exercise into your life

## One Final Thought About The Two Things We All Have in Common

I can't say enough on this simple, unavoidable truth about human physiology:

## We are all designed to move

As my life became more sedentary, I lost sight of this truth, and I lost so much more as well.

Taking the decision to GET MOVING AGAIN had a profound effect on my life. Once I was moving again it just seemed to be most natural thing in the world to explore the second aspect of movement we all have in common.

## We are all designed to work at different metabolic levels

You see, we all have a collection of energy systems. If we lead a sedentary lifestyle these become less efficient. They may even shut down, in the same way that our muscles shut down if we don't use them.

But once you start training to your different metabolic levels, referred to here as Z1, Z2 and Z3, then you start to re-activate your energy systems as well.

I hope you can see that by following the simple Plan outlined in this book you have already started to use **Heart-rated Training** to rebuild your fitness and strength. And by doing so, you have started to reclaim your health too.

So, if you feel you are ready to take things to a completely new level by exercising at **YOUR** different metabolic levels then go for it and.....

## Good luck to you on your journey.

## Follow Our Facebook Page

Even if you are heading off to do your own thing, you can still "Follow Us" via our new Facebook Page where we share updates and training tips, articles from other health & fitness authors and more. You can follow the link here:

https://www.facebook.com/ianbirchwalkruntrain

# 12. RESOURCES

## References

**Ref 1** - Elizabeth Blackburn and Elissa Epel (2017) The Telomere Effect, A revolutionary approach to living younger, healthier, longer. 1st edn. London: Orion Spring

**Ref 2** – Laurence E. Morehouse and Leonard Gross (1977) Total Fitness in 30 minutes a week. 1st edn. Granada Publishing, St Albans

**Ref 3** - Jonathan A. Pye (publisher) and Andrew Hamilton (Editor)(2010) Advanced Fitness Training for elite sports performance. Effective endurance training: why Goldilocks was wrong! London, P2P Publishing

Website:

https://www.sportsperformancebulletin.com

**Ref 4** - Pavel Tsatsouline, Kettlebell Simple & Sinister. Reno, USA, Published by Strongfirst Inc

Website:

https://www.StrongFirst.com

**Ref 5** - Sarah Barker (1978), The Alexander Technique, The revolutionary way to use your body for total energy, Bantam Books, Inc, New York, New York, USA

Also see this great online resource:

The Complete Guide to the Alexander Technique

Website:

https://alexandertechnique.com

## Online Sources

**Source 1** - Comparing Measures of Obesity: Waist Circumference, Waist-Hip, and Waist-Height Ratios.

Alaa Youssef Ahmed Ahmed Baioumi, in Nutrition in the Prevention and Treatment of Abdominal Obesity (Second Edition), 2019

Website: https://www.sciencedirect.com/topics/biochemistry-genetics-and-molecular-biology/waist-to-height-ratio

**Source 2** – Measuring the Waist by The World Cancer Research Fund

Website: https://www.wcrf-uk.org/health-advice-and-support/health-checks/how-to-measure-your-waist/

**Source 3** - The Complete Guide to the Alexander Technique

Your Global Online Resource for the Alexander Technique since 1997:

Website: https://alexandertechnique.com/

# The Power of Walking

Printed in Great Britain
by Amazon

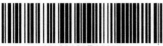

45133630R00057